The Blister Prone Athlete's Guide To Preventing Foot Blisters

Insider Tips To Take You From Blister Victim To Champion

How to stop the 10 most common blisters from heel to toe

Rebecca Rushton BSc(Pod)

© Copyright 2015 Rebecca Rushton trading as
Blister Prevention ABN 74 064 976 429

B/116 Dempster Street,
Esperance WA 6450
Australia
Phone +61 8 9072 1514
Email support@blisterprevention.com.au

The moral rights of the author have been asserted.

All rights reserved. Except under the statutory exceptions provisions of the *Australian Copyright* Act (1968) and for brief extracts for the purposes of review, no part of this book including but not limited to designs in this book may be reproduced, stored or transmitted by any person or entity, including Internet search engines or retailers, in any form or by any means, electronic or mechanical, including photocopying, recording, scanning or by any information storage and retrieval system without the prior written permission of the author.

All the information within this publication is intended to be general information only. The information is not intended to be individual advice, and it is not individual advice. If any reader chooses to make use of the information, it is that reader's decision. It is recommended that the reader obtain his or her own independent professional advice for his or her specific condition. Use of the information in this publication is not intended to create, and does not create, a client or patient relationship between a reader and the author.

The author and publisher have made every effort to ensure that the information in this publication is correct at the time of publication. The author and publisher do not assume and hereby disclaim liability for any injury, loss or damage to persons or property whatsoever, however it may arise, including from negligence or any other cause.

Names of manufacturers, suppliers, business people and products are provided for the information of readers only, with no intention to infringe copyright or trademarks.

Edited by Stephen Lake
Cover design by Karen Phillips
Cover image by Milkwhale Infographics
Printed by CreateSpace POD

First published in 2015.

ISBN: 978-0-646-94357-2

Dedication

This book is dedicated to J Martin Carlson MS, CPO, FAAOP, whose academic research and early mentoring contributed the most to my understanding of shear-related skin injury.

Acknowledgement

To Stephen Lake, whose editing skill and passion knows no bounds, whose wit made writing this book an enjoyable process, and whose kindness will be remembered.

Contents

What you need to know about blisters	1
Friction defined	3
When blister prevention becomes difficult	6
1. Heel blisters - At the back of your heel	8
2. Heel blisters - Edge blisters	12
3. Heel blisters - Under your heel	15
4. Arch blisters	18
5. Blisters under the ball of your foot	21
6. Toe blisters - Under your big toe	26
7. Toe blisters - On the outside of your little toe	30
8. Toe blisters - On the tops of your toes	33
9. Toe blisters - Between your toes	37
10. Toe blisters - On the tips of your toes or under your toenails	43
Summary	49
Glossary	50

What you need to know about blisters

Foot blisters can be tricky to avoid. New shoes, hot days, sweaty feet, hard surfaces, steep hills, longer distances ...

But they don't have to be. With a bit of foot function knowhow, and an understanding of what causes blisters, even the most blister prone athlete can select the right strategy to become blister-free. And if something goes wrong, troubleshooting becomes a straightforward process.

■ Friction blisters only

This book deals with friction blisters on the feet. Blisters from infections (fungal, viral or bacterial), allergies, insect bites and thermal burns are not discussed.

■ But first

Let's clear this up right away. You've probably heard that heat, moisture and friction cause blisters. While these factors are relevant, they are only a small part of the story. The diagram below shows the four factors that combine to cause foot blisters, with all four needed simultaneously to cause a blister.

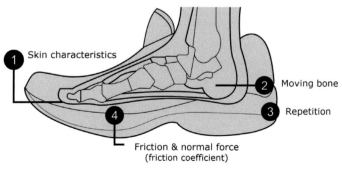

Figure 1: The four factors that combine to provide blister-causing shear.

■ Generally speaking

With the above in mind, we can identify five opportunities for blister prevention success.

1. By gradually increasing the frequency and magnitude of forces applied to the skin, its characteristics change to make it more resistant to blisters. This can be achieved by breaking your shoes in slowly, and progressively increasing your running or walking distance over time. Building thick callous is taking it too far. The changes we're looking for are within the skin layers and not particularly visible.

2. Did you know the foot bones move around quite a lot under the skin? The more they move relative to the skin surface, the more likely you are to get blisters. Changing your biomechanics (the structure and function of your body) in one of several ways can bring immediate blister prevention.

3. If you reduce the number of shear force repetitions to the skin you'll stop blisters. But that means not walking, running or playing so much - not a great option!

4. The coefficient of friction is a ratio of two forces: friction levels (the amount of grip or slipperiness); and normal force (known better as pressure). Both friction and pressure determine the amount of shear that is imparted to the skin. Reduce either and you'll have a direct preventative effect on blisters. I'll expand on this point in a moment - it's super-important.

5. Finally, if you use materials in your shoe that absorb shear, it means the skin then doesn't have to - and that means less blisters. Material selection for socks, insoles and other devices becomes paramount.

Friction defined

Let's get back to number 4 - the coefficient of friction. This needs to be explained because not only is it misunderstood by most people, it is also massively undervalued. Also, I don't want you to take my word for it.

The coefficient of friction is defined by the formula:

$$COF = Friction/Normal\ force$$

Pressure is very relevant to foot blisters because the foot is a weightbearing structure. At the very least, you have weightbearing pressure from standing, walking, running, etc, and contact pressure from your shoe. Then, consider how pressure increases when you add normal bony prominences, abnormal bony deformities, running, jumping, hills, uneven terrain etc.

When it comes to pressure on our feet, in the end, there's only so much we can do. Yes, you could sit out at half time, cut your running distance in half and only hike on flat terrain. And yes, you could have surgery to fix that hammer toe or bunion. But before you have surgery or cut back your activity because of your propensity for blisters, ask yourself this question: "Have I done all I can to minimise friction levels?"

■ Friction - it's not what you think

Friction is good (for the most part). High friction means things grip together. Friction equals traction, with your foot needing traction for the mechanical efficiencies of gait.

Friction is not rubbing! When it comes to blisters, think of friction this way. Shoes, socks and insoles are made of high-friction materials in an attempt to keep your foot still in your shoe. This is both intentional and appropriate. It stops your foot from sliding around in your shoe. But this doesn't stop the bones from moving around inside your foot. Moving bones cause a movement differential to occur between the bone and skin surface. Everything between the bone and skin stretches and distorts. This distortion is called shear, which causes blisters.

■ Blister prone

Most people can tolerate a lot of shear within the skin of their feet. They don't get blisters easily. But some people get blisters very easily - that movement differential between the skin surface and the underlying bone happens to excess (to a level above the shear threshold of our skin) and a blister forms all too quickly. A person's shear threshold is a very individual thing, representing their blister-proneness or blister-resistance.

■ The many faces of friction

When it comes to managing friction to stop blisters, you need to make it more slippery somewhere. This will encourage the movement differential to happen somewhere other than between skin and bone. We're encouraging rubbing - but a safe non-abrasive rubbing!

There are three possible interfaces where the rubbing can occur:

- Between the skin and sock - This is what lubricants do, like Vaseline. Greasy lubricants initially cut friction levels significantly. But as they disperse into the sock and are diluted by sweat, friction levels rise to a level above the baseline level. Either things grip together again, or the rubbing becomes abrasive and damages the skin.

- Between two sock layers - This is what double-socks do. If the friction level between the two socks is lower than on either side (and remains lower in spite of the moisture), rubbing will occur between the sock layers, instead of between skin and bone. Research has shown that double-socks have a moderate effect on reducing blister rates. If you're not particularly blister prone, this could be all it takes to see you blister-free.

- Between the shoe and sock - This is what ENGO Patches do. The friction level at this interface becomes very low because of the patch and remains this low no matter how sweaty the feet or socks get. The sock protects the skin the whole time because there is no rubbing between the two. What's best is you can target blister prone areas only so that traction is maintained everywhere else.

■ Getting traction

Remember how I said traction is important for the mechanical efficiencies of gait? It's very necessary for propulsion and acceleration. It's necessary for efficient deceleration and for rapid changes in direction. Traction is necessary for the efficient transfer of weight from one foot to the next, whether you're walking, running, playing basketball or tennis or football.

Traction stops your toes from jamming into the toe box of your shoe, avoiding black toenails - and worse!

So where do you get traction from? You get traction from high friction levels, from things gripping together.

So friction is good, but it can be bad when we get blisters. The important thing to realise is that friction is necessary and is why your shoes, socks and insoles are made out of high-friction materials. It's only when high friction levels are giving you blisters that you need to manage that friction – and only in that discrete location. Not all over, just in the area of your blisters so you can maintain necessary traction.

When blister prevention becomes difficult

Sometimes it can feel like you've tried everything but you still get blisters and you have no idea why. If you need to get serious about your blisters, this book is for you. If you're tired of stuffing around with things that don't work. If you want to save time and money on what won't work. If you want to cut to the chase and get on top of foot blisters for good ... this book is for you. Regardless of your activity or environmental conditions, successful blister prevention is possible for even the most blister prone person.

■ In this book

I'm going to get specific because that's the direction blister prevention needs to move if it's to be useful to anyone who is blister prone. You'll be getting insider tips from someone who knows what it's like to suffer with blisters in sport. Who specialises in dealing with blisters in the athletic arena. And who knows about feet and how they work.

This book has advice on the ten most common blister locations on the feet. For each blister location, I'll be explaining the anatomical and biomechanical reasons for blisters. I'll show you specific prevention strategies that work best (in no particular order), based on those reasons. I'll include the pros and cons to help you choose the strategy that suits you most, and most likely to work for the blister prone athlete. Some of these strategies are straight-forward and you can institute them yourself. Others are a little more involved and you may need to seek professional help. The point is, they're the most applicable to that anatomical location and most likely to work for the blister prone athlete.

■ A certain amount will be assumed

I won't be explaining general blister prevention advice. The following will be assumed:

- You've attempted to train your skin to the loads it will be enduring, benefitting from the adaptive skin changes that can be the difference between blisters and no blisters.
- You're wearing shoes that are appropriate to the activity and that fit perfectly.
- If appropriate, you're wearing moisture-wicking socks in an effort to minimise the increased friction effect of the sweaty shoe environment.
- Cutting back on your activity is an obvious blister prevention strategy, but one that is generally unacceptable and will not be considered.

Please note that this book has general information on friction blister management only, and is not a substitute for medical or professional care. If you believe you have any other health problem, or if you have any questions regarding your health or a medical condition, you should promptly consult your physician or other healthcare provider.

1 Heel blisters - At the back of your heel

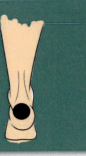

■ Cause

The Achilles tendon attaches to the back of the heel bone (calcaneus). The anatomy and function of these structures can lead to heel blisters in two ways:

- As we walk and run, the calcaneus is pulled upwards by tension in the Achilles. This biomechanical function is normal. However, if the calf muscles are tight, extra tension in the tendon causes the calcaneus to lift sooner, higher and with more force. That can be a problem when it happens in the presence of high friction levels, which as I've explained, is a given.
- Some people have a bony lump at the back of the heel called a Haglund's deformity. In this situation, pressure is much higher on the skin. When combined with high friction levels, shear distortions are more likely to be blister-causing.

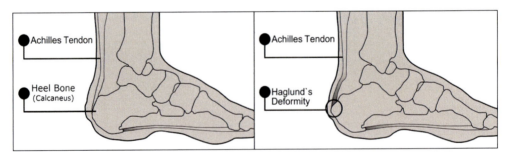

Figure 2: Normal and abnormal anatomy at the back of the heel.

■ Prevention

As a long-time heel blister sufferer myself, there are five prevention strategies worth considering.

1 Lacing

Holding your heel down in your shoe will help to minimise abrasive rubbing. It might not be enough to stop blisters, because this doesn't stop the movement differential between skin and bone. But it can provide significant relief. Adjusting your laces is something you can do on the fly - if you don't have time to stop for too long, or you don't have access to your blister kit (you have a blister kit, right?). The Lace-Lock (Heel-Lock) lacing technique is the best lacing technique to keep your heel secured firmly. You use the last eyelet on your shoes to make a loop on either side, feed each lace through the opposite loop, pull them firmly (down), and then tie your normal bow.

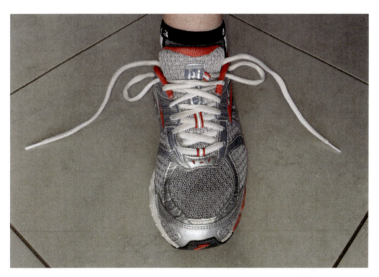

Figure 3: The Lace-Lock (Heel-Lock) lacing technique.

2 Calf Stretch

You can reduce tension in the Achilles tendon by stretching the calf muscles. There are two muscles so two stretches are needed. Stretching is almost always overlooked and could hold the key for getting rid of your heel blisters. It takes weeks to see the results, so it's something to do well before you get blisters. See your podiatrist to make sure you're doing these stretches correctly and that they are appropriate for you. While you're there, your podiatrist might consider other treatments like heel lifts, joint mobilisations or other therapies.

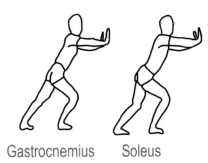

Figure 4: Calf stretching reduces tension in the Achilles tendon.

3 ENGO Patches

ENGO Patches are the best way to reduce friction levels at the back of the heel. They're better than lubricants because they keep friction levels low indefinitely and they last for months. Another difference is they encourage the movement differential between your shoe and sock. In this way, there is no chance of abrasive rubbing on your skin. ENGO Patches work best preventively, but they'll also provide significant relief when used in blister treatment.

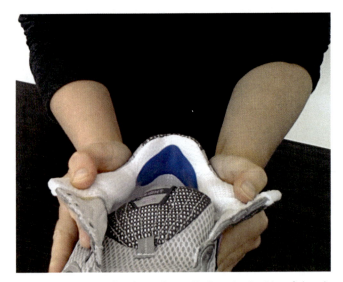

Figure 5: Blue ENGO heel patch applied to the inside of the shoe.

4 Taping and Dressings

Taping provides a protective layer to the skin that can help protect against the abrasive effect of your sock and any grit that gets into your shoe. Unfortunately, taping doesn't always stop blisters. Depending on the friction properties of the tape, its rigidity and thickness, blister-causing shear can still occur underneath it.

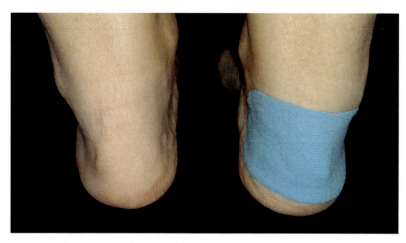

Figure 6: Taping provides a protective layer to the skin.

5 Donut Pads

While more useful as a blister treatment, donut pads can be used preventively. To make a donut pad, cut a hole in a piece of thick orthopaedic felt or moleskin and place it so the blister area is in the hole. The donut pad lifts the shoe off the blister to provide some pressure relief. You'll need to put tape over the donut pad to keep it in place for any length of time.

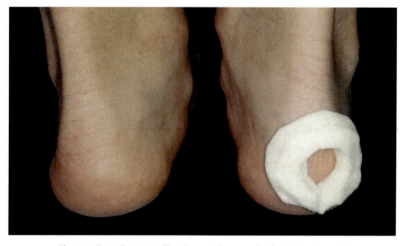

Figure 7: A 7 mm adhesive orthopaedic felt donut pad.

2 Heel blisters - Edge blisters

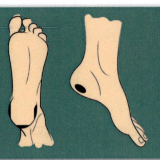

■ Cause

Edge blisters can occur around the heel's rim. They're caused by an irritation to the skin where the insole or orthotic meets the side of the shoe. As the blister fills with more fluid, weightbearing pressure pushes the blister fluid upwards. It can trick you into thinking the blister is caused by something higher up the side of the heel.

■ Prevention

Prevention of edge blisters at the heel is all about two things: pressure from the heel cup of the insole or orthotic; and friction levels at that junction.

1 Eliminate excess pressure from the heel cup

- Insole: Your insole's curved heel cup may be creased or buckled or protrude into your skin in some way. If you can't position it so the contour of the heel cup blends seamlessly with the side of the shoe, replace it with a new one.

- Orthotic: If your orthotic has slipped forward, you'll be standing on the heel cup, with blisters (or at least callouses) a certainty. Apply some double-sided tape under the orthotic and fix it so it's sitting correctly at the back of your shoe. Another cause of blisters is a thick or misshapen heel cup. Your podiatrist will be able to adjust this by either heat-moulding or grinding it.

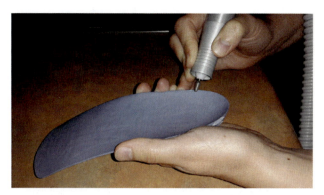

Figure 8: A podiatrist can grind the inside of the heel cup to make it less of an irritation.

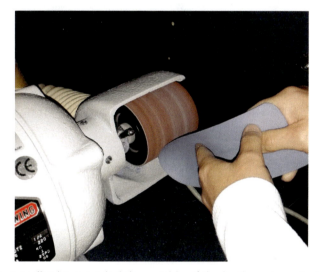

Figure 9: A podiatrist can grind the outside of the heel cup to make it thinner.

2 Making a low-friction junction

With the heel cup of your insole or orthotic sorted out, if you're still getting edge blisters, you'll need to manage friction with ENGO Patches. This will create a low-friction junction between the shoe and the heel cup. Cover each surface with a separate large oval patch using the Two-Patch Technique: one patch goes on the shoe, the other on the insole or orthotic.

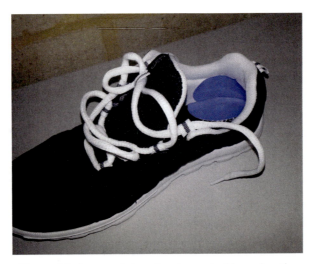

Figure 10: A smooth junction is created by using the Two-Patch Technique with ENGO Patches.

To get the Two-Patch Technique right for the heel, you need to make sure of two things:

- The top rim of the heel cup is covered with the patch (so make sure this is where the widest part of the patch is); and
- There are no creases that will irritate the skin. Creases on the outside of the heel cup are fine and in fact are usually necessary on curved and contoured heel cups.

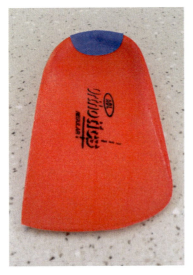

Figure 11: Make sure the widest part of the patch goes over the heel cup.

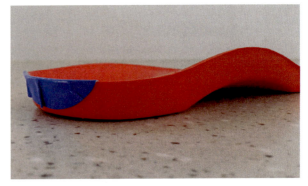

Figure 12: For edge blisters at the back of the heel, creases on the outside of the heel cup are fine.

3 Heel blisters - Under your heel

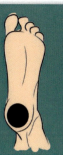

■ Cause

Blisters under the heel are most often suffered by hikers and runners on downhill terrain. These blisters are painful and difficult to treat, which makes prevention all the more important.

■ Prevention

1 Change your gait

If possible, the best preventative strategy for blisters under your heel is to alter your gait. The following will help. Please keep in mind that these compensations may have a detrimental effect elsewhere and must be implemented gradually:

- Avoiding a heel strike and opting for more of a midfoot or forefoot initial contact;
- Making your heel strike more underneath you rather than out in front;
- More knee and hip flexion; and
- A shorter stride length.

2 Lace firmly

Make sure your laces are tied firmly. If that's not enough to stop your foot from sliding forward in your shoe, use the Lace-Lock (Heel-Lock) lacing technique. After making a loop on each side using the last eyelet, take each lace through the opposite loop, pull down to tighten, then tie your normal knot and bow.

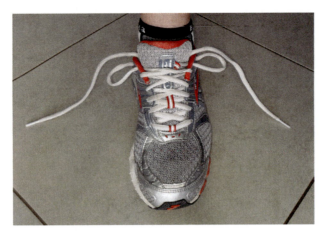

Figure 13: The Lace-Lock (Heel-Lock) lacing technique.

3 Heel cushions

Cushioning under the heel will reduce pressure and absorb some of the shear that otherwise causes a blister. If some shear is absorbed by the cushioning material, less shear will occur within your skin. If your current insole is thin under the heel, consider replacing it. Or you can use a cushion only under the heels (pictured below). Be sure to have one in both shoes so you don't create the effect of having one leg longer than the other.

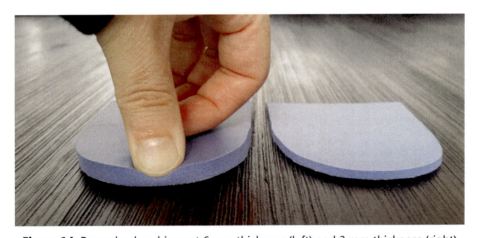

Figure 14: Poron heel cushions at 6 mm thickness (left) and 3 mm thickness (right)

I don't recommend silicone gel materials for cushioning under the heel, even though they provide very good cushioning. The reason for this is they are too good at absorbing shear. Your foot will lose traction as soon as it contacts the ground, compromising your balance and predisposing you to injury. Conversely, there's no point using foam that's too flimsy which neither cushions nor absorbs shear. It can be a fine line, so see your podiatrist if you're not sure what to use.

4 ENGO Patches

If changing your running or walking style is insufficient, you've got a bit of cushioning under your heel and you've got your foot firmly secured in your shoe with lacing, you'll need to reduce friction levels. Do this with an ENGO Patch. You could cover the whole heel area of your insole with a rectangle patch. But more than any other part of the gait cycle, the foot needs a bit of traction when it first hits the ground. Without it, your balance and stability will be compromised. So if you can possibly get away with it, use a small oval patch to cover only the area that requires protection.

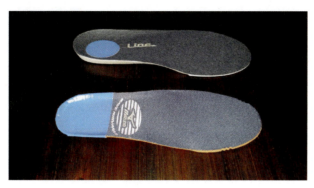

Figure 15: ENGO Patches under the heel - Small oval (top); rectangle with excess folded over (below).

5 Taping

You could try taping your heels. I suggest using a rigid (non-stretch) sports tape. That way it will help distribute the shear load over a larger area. It might not be enough to stop the blister from forming, but it will at least help keep any blister roof intact.

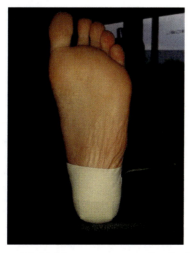

Figure 16: Rigid sports tape under the heel.

4 Arch blisters

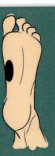

■ Cause

Arch blisters can occur with shoes with a higher arch contour or with the use of orthotics. Relevant factors to consider are:
- You're making a relatively non-weightbearing area of skin more weightbearing;
- The orthotic edge where it abuts the side of the shoe may be causing an edge blister;
- The support provided by the orthotic might be inadequate; and
- The arch contour of the orthotic may be too high.

■ Prevention

1 Condition your skin

If your shoes are more supportive in the arch than you're used to, or you've just started wearing orthotics, all of a sudden the skin will be subjected to weightbearing forces it's not used to. Given time, it will toughen a little as it gets used to dealing with this shear. This will go at least some way to protecting against blisters.

2 ENGO Patches

You can put an ENGO Patch on the arch of your insole, orthotic or shoe to let the sock glide over it. By reducing the friction level like this, the small but early glide stops the shear that causes blisters. Use the Two-Patch Technique if your blister extends to the side of your arch, called an edge blister. The Two-Patch technique for edge blisters involves putting one patch on the orthotic and one patch on the side of the shoe.

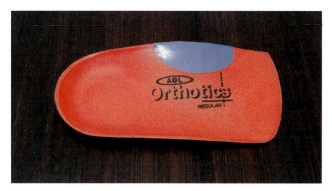

Figure 17: ENGO Patch for arch blisters.

3 Reduce arch height (and maybe cushioning)

To reduce localised pressure, your podiatrist may lower the arch height of your orthotic, reduce its stiffness or change the arch contour in some way. Alternatively, a cushioned orthotic cover might be added. This will not only reduce pressure but will also absorb a bit of shear. Some materials work better than others at this. But as a DIY option, if your orthotic has no cover on it and you feel like you need a bit of cushioning or shear absorption, if the shoe's insole is flat and non-contoured, you could try putting it on top of your orthotic.

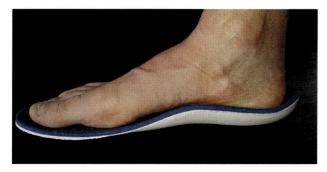

Figure 18: Orthotics with a high arch height and cushioned cover.

4 Change the orthotic so it supports the foot better

You can also get arch blisters when the arch contour of your orthotic is too low; or the overall functional support it provides is inadequate. An important function of the foot regarding arch blisters is the windlass mechanism, which prepares your foot for effective propulsion. When ineffective or absent, the arch does not elevate on its own as your weight moves from heel to toe. Your podiatrist can do something about that. There are several orthotic design features that can reduce the force needed to engage the windlass mechanism, and to help the mechanism kick in earlier. These design features can go a long way to preventing arch blisters.

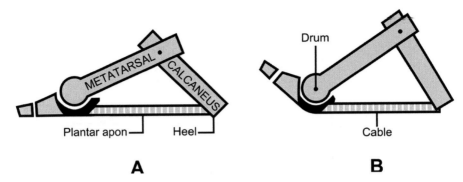

Figure 19: The windlass mechanism is an important consideration for arch blisters.

5 Blisters under the ball of your foot

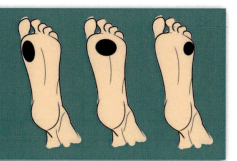

■ Cause

The ball of the foot is an important weightbearing area of the foot. When the forefoot plants, the underlying metatarsal bones skid forward over the skin, and then backwards during propulsion. All the soft tissue in between is compressed and stretched. It's easy to imagine the shear that occurs in this area of the foot. It's normal, it happens with every step we take and our skin is able to deal with a lot of it. But it can become excessive under certain scenarios, including:

1. One of the metatarsal bones protrudes more than the others;
2. Your foot works in a way that means load distribution is uneven;
3. Tight calf muscles cause more load under the ball of the foot region;
4. You're wearing shoes with a thin sole or with no cushioning insole; and
5. The fatty padding under the ball of your foot becomes thinner (some people have less of this natural cushioning than others, and it reduces with age).

■ Prevention

1 Cushioned insoles

Cushioning has a double blister prevention effect:

- It reduces peak pressure (some materials cushion better than others); and
- It absorbs some shear. That is, shear occurs within the material so less of it occurs within your skin.

Adding cushioned insoles can be an easy change to make, especially if your current insoles are flimsy or compressed. Podiatrists use materials like Spenco and Poron for insoles and orthotic covers to reduce pressure and absorb shear. I do not recommend silicone gel materials under the ball of the foot, even though they provide very good cushioning. The reason is they are exceptionally good at absorbing shear, so much so that they severely diminish traction. This has ramifications for your balance and propulsive efficiency. Save silicone gel materials for toe blisters where traction is not so critical!

Blisters can still form in spite of cushioning. That's because the friction levels of most cushioning materials are high. So if you're still getting blisters in spite of cushioned insoles, consider adding the next strategy on top of your insoles to address high friction levels.

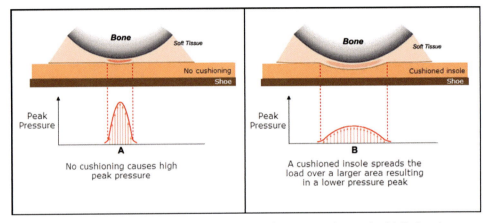

Figure 20: The effect of cushioning on peak pressure (image by M Carlson).

2 ENGO Patches

ENGO Patches reduce friction really well. Pictured are the large ovals - the best way to target most blister areas. If you need broader protection, you can use the larger rectangle patches. Remember, the ball of the foot is an important weightbearing area that needs friction for traction. Unless you are getting blisters across the whole ball of the foot, first try a large oval, or cut a rectangle patch down to size. A targeted approach to friction management is always better than reducing friction levels all over.

ENGO Patches do not reduce pressure (at 0.38 mm thick, it's important to note they don't increase pressure either). They work entirely by reducing friction levels. To have the best of both worlds, add an ENGO Patch to your cushioned insole and benefit from both pressure and friction management.

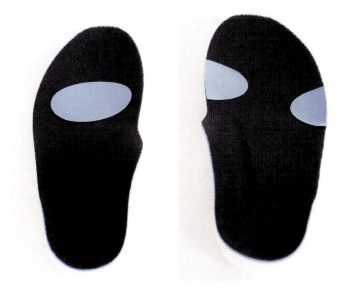

Figure 21: Large oval ENGO Patches under the ball of the foot.

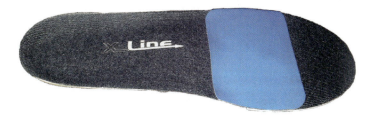

Figure 22: Rectangle ENGO Patch under the ball of the foot.

3 Taping

Applying tape to the ball of the foot will do two things:

- It will negate the abrasive effect of your sock, sand and grit against your skin; and
- If it's a rigid (non-stretch) tape, it will help to spread shear load over a wider area.

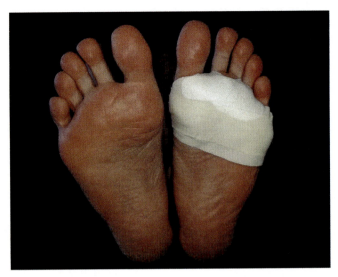

Figure 23: Taping under the ball of the foot.

4 Donut pads

Donut pads are another way to reduce pressure at blister prone areas. Whilst the downside is that they're quite bulky, donut pads come into their own as a blister treatment. When you've got a blister, the skin is weak, and considering that you have to walk on the ball of the foot, taking some pressure off it will be a priority. You'll need to put tape over the donut pad to keep it in place for any length of time.

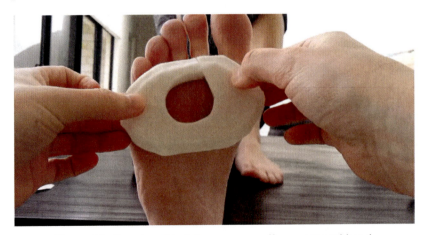

Figure 24: Donut pad to take pressure off a metatarsal head.

5 Biomechanical improvements

Blisters under the ball of the foot are often associated with structural and biomechanical issues. There's a lot that a podiatrist can do to alter your biomechanics to reduce the incidence of blisters at this part of your foot. This could involve insoles, orthotics, stretches, joint mobilisations or modifications in your gait or running style. It all depends on your individual biomechanical needs. If you're not getting anywhere with your blister prevention efforts, see your podiatrist.

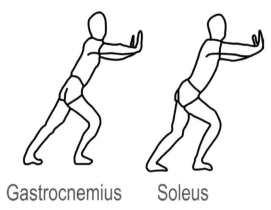

Figure 25: A calf stretching regime can help to reduce the duration and magnitude of load across the ball of the foot.

6 Toe blisters - Under your big toe

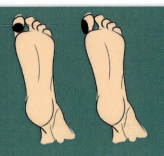

■ Cause

Blisters under the big toe are more than likely a consequence of your foot's structure or biomechanics. Here are some potential causes:

- You walk with your feet turned out and roll off the side of your big toe rather than toeing-off straight through the toe.
- Your big toe is angled towards the other toes (often the result of a bunion) and you roll off the side of the toe rather than toeing-off straight through the toe.
- You're wearing shoes that are too narrow at the toes, so a part of your big toe is "hanging over the edge" of the shoe.
- Your big toe knuckle is stiff in the upwards direction causing higher weightbearing forces under the big toe.
- Your big toe is turned up at the end causing higher pressure under the middle of the big toe.

■ Prevention

1 Dealing with the biomechanics

If you're getting blisters under your big toe, you need to see a podiatrist, who is best placed to understand the mechanical reasons behind them. The most common biomechanical issue that predisposes to blisters under your big toe is an inefficient windlass mechanism. The windlass mechanism is an important biomechanical function in the foot that promotes efficient gait. When this is not working efficiently, one consequence is high pressure under the big toe.

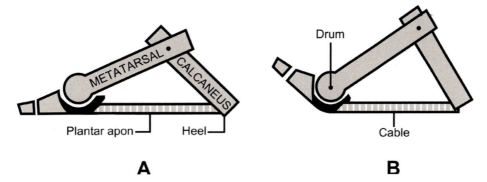

Figure 26: A functional hallux limitus is a result of an inefficient windlass mechanism. It causes more pressure under the big toe.

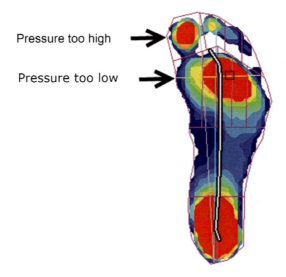

Figure 27: The pressure map of a runner with a functional hallux limitus. Blue indicates low pressure and red indicates high pressure.

Take a look at the pressure map above. This represents a "functional hallux limitus". This is caused by an inefficient windlass mechanism, which means there is plenty of upwards bend at the big toe knuckle when non-weightbearing, but not when walking. The result is an excessive amount of pressure borne by the big toe. In most circumstances this is easily fixed with orthotics with very specific design features.

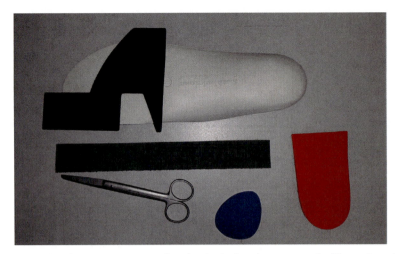

Figure 28: Podiatrists can use several orthotic design features to facilitate the windlass mechanism so load is reduced under the big toe.

But sometimes this limited motion is a structural bony restriction, which means it can't be fixed without surgical intervention. Your podiatrist will identify what's going on with your feet and give you advice specific to your situation.

2 ENGO Patches

Don't forget to address friction. Especially if changing your foot function is insufficient, you'll need to rely on reducing friction levels. This is best done with ENGO Patches because you can target this area only and leave traction unaffected everywhere else. If the blistering is just under the toe, a patch under the toe is all that's needed (pictured below). If you're dealing with more of an edge blister, use the Two-Patch Technique. This is where you apply another patch to the side of the shoe, on the inside of the toe box. Don't underestimate the ability of this technique to stop these blisters.

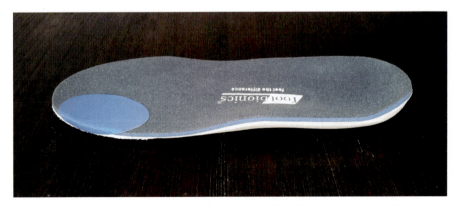

Figure 29: ENGO Patch (large oval) placement for blisters under the big toe.

3 Silicone gel toe sleeve

If neither of these provide sufficient blister prevention, use a silicone gel toe sleeve to cushion the toe and absorb a good deal of the shear. There are two potential downsides to consider, however. The first is the lack of traction under the big toe. This may or may not have on an adverse effect on your propulsive efficiency. The second is skin maceration. Silicone gel toe sleeves prevent the evaporation of moisture and can cause the skin to become uncomfortably hot, sweaty and soggy. Some people can wear them for extended periods without issue; others aren't so fortunate. An open-ended silicone gel toe sleeve would be preferable to one that is closed-in at the end as it gives sweat another escape route. A closed-in silicone gel toe cap is only necessary when protection is needed for the tip of the toe.

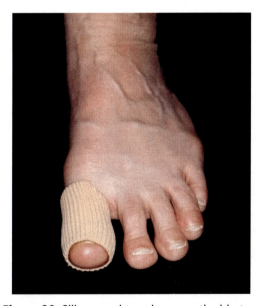

Figure 30: Silicone gel toe sleeve on the big toe.

7 Toe blisters - On the outside of your little toe

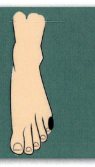

■ Cause

Blisters on the outside of the little toe are possibly the most common toe blisters. The dominant cause is when the toe curls and tucks in and under the next one, making the joints more prominent. Just like your little finger, there are three bones in your little toe. When it bends and twists, the two joints become prominent and susceptible to blisters.

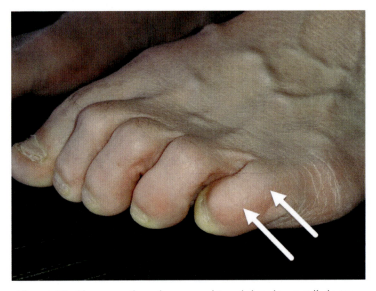

Figure 31: There are three bones and two joints in your little toe.

■ Prevention

There are three prevention strategies I advise for blisters on the outside of the little toe.

1 Shoe fit

As mentioned in the introduction, it was assumed that you were already wearing perfectly fitting shoes, and this factor is paramount for avoiding blisters on the outside of the little toe. Here are a few things to keep in mind:

- The shoe toe box depth and width simply must accommodate your toes. You can't expect to be pain-free or blister-free without this important aspect of shoe fit being met.
- Tie your laces firmly to prevent your foot slipping forward and jamming your toes into a narrower part of the toe box.
- Shoes with a more flexible upper in the region of the little toe will help.
- Seams in the shoe's upper will make the situation worse.

Unfortunately, even with all of these aspects of shoe fit being met, blisters on the outside of the little toes are still possible. Why? Because we haven't fixed the root of the problem - the curly toe. There are two more things you can try, to address the pressure and friction that contribute to blister-causing shear.

2 Silicone gel toe sleeve

These devices are great for two reasons:

1. They cushion the prominent joints, reducing pressure; and
2. The silicone material is excellent at absorbing shear. And remember, the more shear that occurs within the silicone, the less shear will be happening within the skin of your little toe.

The silicone gel toe devices limit the evaporation of moisture, however, and this can make the skin between the toes macerated if worn for extended periods. Use a closed-in silicone gel toe cap, like the one pictured below, if you need protection near the tip of the toe. Otherwise, an open-ended silicone gel toe sleeve will be adequate. Additionally, the open ended sleeve will allow sweat to drain from both ends to reduce maceration. If maceration is an issue for you, you could tape the toe. While tape won't absorb any shear and may not reduce friction levels, it will protect the skin from abrasive rubbing.

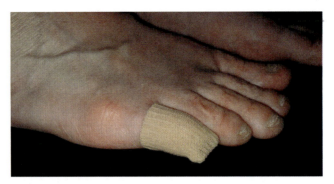

Figure 32: This is a silicone gel toe cap (it's closed in at the end). You could also use the silicone gel toe sleeves that are open at the end.

3 ENGO Patches

An ENGO Patch is a great way to reduce friction levels in this location. Consider it if the silicone gel toe cover takes up too much room in your shoe or if it causes too much maceration. Note that if you're wearing shoes with mesh uppers, water can get in from the outside. This may render the adhesive ineffective and the patch may dislodge.

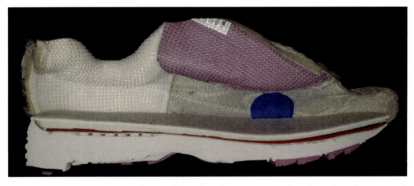

Figure 33: An ENGO Patch on the inside of a shoe upper. The shoe has been cut in half.

8 Toe blisters - On the tops of your toes

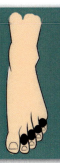

■ Cause

Clawed toes and hammer toes make the toe joints sit up higher and are hence more susceptible to blisters. This can be a structural thing - the toes are fixed in this position. Or it can be a functional thing - the toes are perfectly able to straighten, but when you walk and run, they bend over.

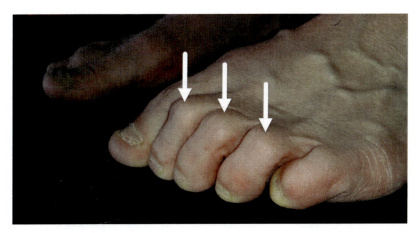

Figure 34: Clawed toes with prominent toe joints.

■ Prevention

1 Shoe toe box depth

Let's talk shoe fit again, specifically for these blisters:
- The toe box depth simply must accommodate your toes. You can't expect to be pain-free or blister-free without this important aspect of shoe fit being met.
- Tie your laces firmly to prevent your foot slipping forward into a shallower part of the toe box.

- Shoes with a more flexible upper in the toe box region will help.
- Seams across the prominent toe joints are going to make this worse.

2 Change toe posture

The toes can adopt a clawed posture for a number of reasons. If it's a fixed deformity, you'll need to hope that the other options explained here do the trick. Otherwise, your only option might be to have the toes surgically straightened. If your toes can straighten, a podiatrist may be able to do something to encourage your toes to maintain this straighter posture. This could involve orthotics, stretches, toe devices or other treatments. Toe props can be used to take up the space under the toes and prevent them bending over so much. While the toe prop is in place, the toes will sit straighter, making the joints on top less prominent. Athletes should experiment with these to ensure the material between the toes doesn't irritate in any way, particularly over long distances.

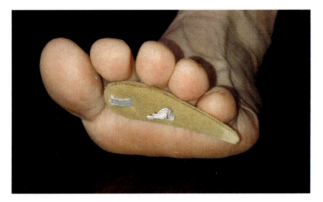

Figure 35: Off-the-shelf toe prop (elastic over the toe to hold it in place).

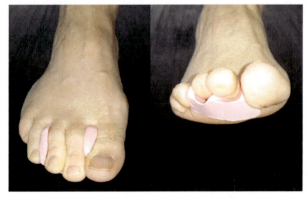

Figure 36: Custom-made toe prop (held in place with contouring and apposition of toes).

3 Taping

The skin on the top of the toes is easily abraded if it rubs against the top of the toe box. Tape can provide a protective layer to minimise that rubbing, helping to stop abrasions and blisters. Although a non-stretch tape will help distribute shear load better, a stretchy tape is easier to apply without leaving creases - it's difficult but important for this area. A good technique (one that is most likely to stay intact) involves closing in the end of the toe. Take one piece of tape over the toe from bottom to top, and another around the toe so the tape ends meet at the top of the toe.

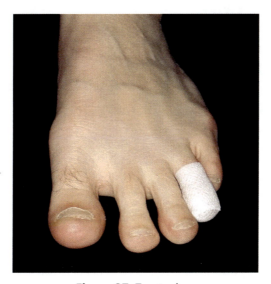

Figure 37: Toe taping.

4 Silicone gel toe sleeve

A silicone toe cover will both cushion the prominent joints and absorb a large amount of the shear. These devices are a little bulky, so it could get tricky if you need protection for two or more toes on the same foot - there might not be enough room in your toe box to accommodate them. Whether you choose a silicone gel toe sleeve (open at the end) or silicone gel toe cap (closed in at the end) is up to you. Considering your blister is on the top of the toe, you only need the open-ended sleeve, like the one pictured below. Being open at both ends will have the added advantage that sweat can escape from both ends, minimising the chance of skin maceration. But if your toe is bent over and you'd also like to protect the tip of the toe, consider a closed-in cap.

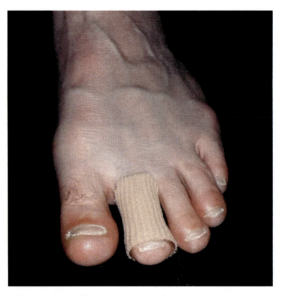

Figure 38: Silicone gel toe sleeve (open at end).

5 ENGO Blister Prevention Patch

When silicone covers are not an option, an ENGO Patch applied to the inside of the toe box is an excellent way to reduce friction levels at the tops of the toes. This is especially the case if you feel like you've done everything you can with shoe fit and the posture of your toes. Remember that if your shoe upper is permeable to water, the patch could dislodge if it gets too wet.

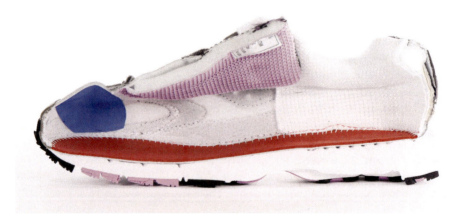

Figure 39: An ENGO large oval patch on the inner toe box of the shoe to protect against blisters on top of the toes. The shoe has been cut in half.

9 Toe blisters - Between your toes

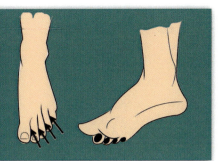

■ Cause

There are two types of interdigital blisters:
- True interdigital blisters - blisters literally between two toes.
- Pinch blisters - blisters towards the bottom or end of the toe. Pinch blisters are common with curly toes. As one toe sits under the next, the toe underneath gets trodden on with each step. This pinching causes the soft tissue of the toe to become a triangular shape and there is often a ridge of callous.

Toes are bony little things. There are three phalanges (toe bones) in each toe (except the big toe which has two, like your thumb). Phalanges aren't smooth straight bones, they're pretty lumpy. Look at the X-ray below of the big toe and second toe. In this image you can see the soft tissue of each toe and even the nails if you look closely. And you can see the phalanges under the skin. Notice how they are wide at the ends and skinny in the middle. Even at the best of times, you can see how the bony prominence of one toe can press on the bony prominence of an adjacent toe. This is even more so when a toe is bent or curly.

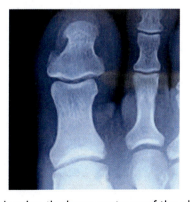

Figure 40: An X-ray showing the bony anatomy of the phalanges (toe bones) of the big toe and second toe.

■ Prevention

1 Silicone gel toe sleeves, caps and wedges

Silicone gel toe sleeves, caps and wedges are used to:

- Cushion bony prominences via the bulk of the material;
- Keep the toes physically separated; and
- Absorb shear.

The open-ended sleeves are good because they are elasticised sufficiently to stay on the toe and provide 360 degree protection. The closed-in caps (not pictured) are also elasticised and will have the added benefit of blister protection right to the tip of the toe. The wedges are thicker and offer more cushioning and shear absorption. However, the only thing holding them in place is the toes themselves, so they can dislodge.

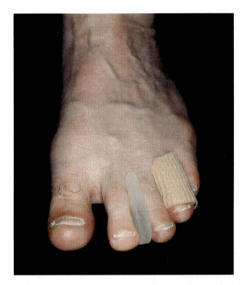

Figure 41: Silicone gel toe sleeves and interdigital wedges for blisters between toes.

Some people find that silicone devices make the skin too sweaty. This is a very individual issue and I have seen both sides of the coin: continual wear over a six-day ultramarathon without any problems; to significant skin maceration and an intolerable feeling of heat after a couple of hours at rest. You won't know until you experiment with them. I highly recommend them as worth trying for most toe blisters, particularly interdigital blisters.

2 Custom-made interdigital wedge/separator

Podiatrists use a mouldable putty material that sets and holds its shape. We use it frequently to make wedges to achieve an even pressure along the entire interdigital space, in spite of the most significant toe deformities. It's the best way to reduce pressure - better than cushioning methods (above). However, it isn't always tolerated because it can feel hard and foreign in some cases. It's worth a try though, especially if other strategies don't help enough. The aim is either to get the toe to sit straighter, or if not, at least prevent high focal pressure by moulding the material to the interdigital space. Because non-weightbearing toe alignment is always different to weightbearing toe alignment, you need to be standing while the material sets. The good thing about this material is that it's long-lasting (at least months) and is easy to keep clean.

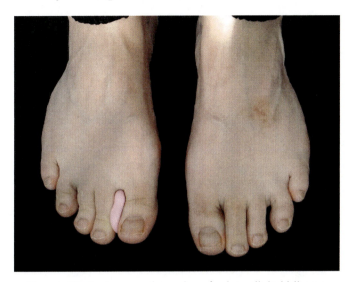

Figure 42: Custom-made wedges for interdigital blisters.

3 Taping

Tapes or dressings can be used to:
- Reposition a toe;
- Encapsulate the soft tissue of the toe; and
- Protect the skin from abrasive rubbing.

Taping can reposition a bent toe so it sits a little straighter. For example, if you have a curly toe that tucks "in and under" the next toe, use the tape to pull the toe in the opposite direction - "up and out". Depending on the degree of the deformity and the amount of tension you exert on the tape, this may not be comfortable for long periods. On the other hand, tape stretches and/or comes loose over time so depending on your activity it needs to be replaced each day, or several times a day.

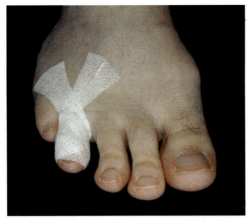

Figure 43: Tape can be used to hold a bent toe in a different position.

For toes that suffer pinch blisters, the fleshy underside of the toe is often misshapen to the point where it can be triangular. Tape can retain this soft tissue, amounting to less pinching of that flesh by the next toe. This alone can significantly help prevent pinch blisters.

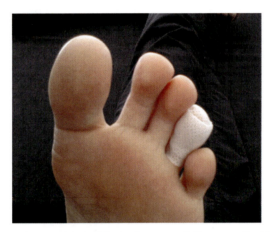

Figure 44: Tape can be used to hold misshapen soft tissue so that less of this skin is pinched by the adjacent toe.

4 Lubricants

Lubricants reduce friction and can be worth a try for blisters between your toes. However, after a while friction increases. So to remain successful, reapplication is required, otherwise, you're actually more likely to get blisters. Also, lubricants lock sweat within the skin and can increase maceration. On the upside, if used only between the toes, at least the initial lack of traction will be a minor issue at this anatomical location. Vaseline is an example of a greasy lubricant; talcum powder is an example of a lubricant in powdered form. There are many more complex lubricants on the market.

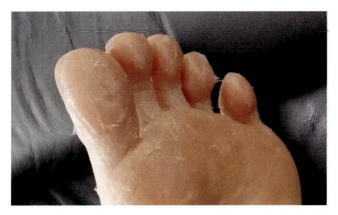

Figure 45: Vaseline applied to the foot for preventing blisters. For interdigital blisters, use only between the toes, not all over the forefoot like this.

5 Toe socks

Toe socks work in three ways:

- They're a double-sock system by forming an additional interface (a sock-sock interface) at the interdigital space.
- They add a little more bulk to the interdigital space to cushion the area.
- This bulk acts to absorb some shear.

Toe socks may be all you need to stop blisters from forming between your toes. I recommend them as a good starting point. While toe socks can reduce interdigital blisters, it's not difficult to understand how they can cause the shoe to get too tight in the toe box and cause additional pressure and more blisters to the outside of the big and little toes.

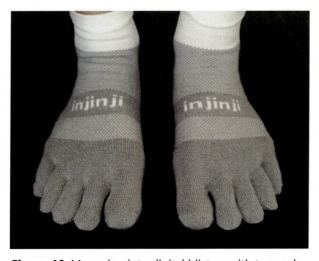

Figure 46: Managing interdigital blisters with toe socks.

6 ENGO Patches on toe socks

Applying an ENGO Patch to toe socks reduces friction a lot more than the toe socks alone. In the picture below, I've cut a rectangle patch into strips. As you wrap the patch around the toe, in case your feet swell, take care not to apply compression. Just lay it on and press to adhere. By applying one strip to each of the second and fourth toes, there's protection for all interdigital spaces, avoiding the need for ENGO on every toe. This is a great way to reduce friction levels. The only problem is it won't last like ENGO on the shoe or insole does because unfortunately, it won't survive a soapy washing machine cycle. But if you find yourself in a tricky situation and you need a quick and effective fix to see you through, this will provide significant relief.

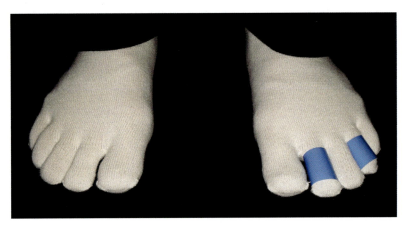

Figure 47: ENGO Patches on toe socks

10 Toe blisters - On the tips of your toes or under your toenails

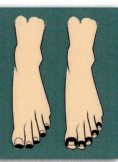

■ Cause

Pressure is the predominant cause of these blisters, with friction playing a secondary part.

Pressure could be coming from:

- Thickened rough toenails catching on socks or shoe seams.
- Swelling can make an otherwise well-fitting shoe too small.
- Toes that are bent over (clawed or hammer toes), causing the tip of the toe and toenail to sustain weightbearing pressure.
- Your toes hitting the end of your shoe, pushing your nail back into the toe repeatedly.

Toenails are attached to the skin underneath them, the nail bed. When you push your toenail from the end, it pulls on this nail bed, and shear occurs within the nail bed skin layers.

■ Prevention

1 Shoe fit

Shoes that are too small mean that your toes hit against the end of the shoe. Shoes that are too big mean that your foot can slide forward and hit the end of the shoe. Both scenarios are equally bad, although at least with shoes that are too big you can make use of firm lacing techniques to keep the foot positioned correctly in the shoe. To determine whether your shoe is the right length, ensure you have the width of your thumb between the end of your longest toe and the end of the upper, measured when you are standing.

2 Cutting and filing nails

Long, thick and rough nails will very likely lead to toenail blisters and in most cases are simple to avoid. Do your best to file the nails down. If you can't seem to get anywhere with your nails, see a podiatrist - we have a machine that painlessly thins even the thickest nails. If there's something more complicated going on (nail or toe deformities), a podiatrist can advise you on other options.

3 Change toe posture

Toe props can be used to prevent blisters on the tips of the toes and around the toenails when clawed or hammer toes are causing these blisters. The aim is to stop you from walking on the tips of the toes, or at least to lessen the weightbearing pressure. Toe props take up the space under your toes and encourage your toes to sit straighter. Toe props can be purchased pre-made, or custom-made.

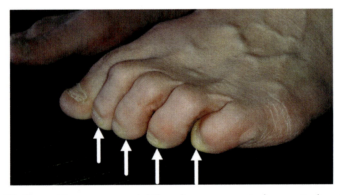

Figure 48: Clawed toes cause weightbearing pressure to be exerted on the end of the toes and toenails.

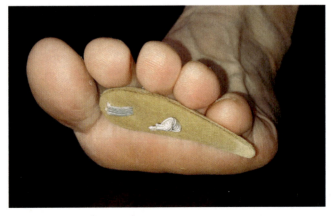

Figure 49: Off-the-shelf toe prop (elastic over the toe to hold it in place).

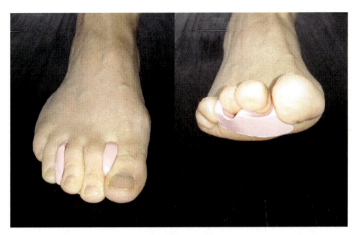

Figure 50: Custom-made toe prop (held in place with contouring and apposition of toes).

Toe props can be great for everyday use and they last a long time (at least months - for the custom-made ones). Long-distance runners and hikers will need to experiment to ensure the toe props are suitable for long durations.

4 ENGO Patches

Assuming your toes are clawed or hammered, if toe props don't work and your shoe toe box is as deep as possible, apply an ENGO patch to the insole. This will minimise friction levels and help prevent blisters on the tips of the toes, not so much under the toenails. If it's the majority of your toes, use a rectangle patch and trim off the excess (pictured below). If it's one or two toes, an oval patch might provide adequate coverage.

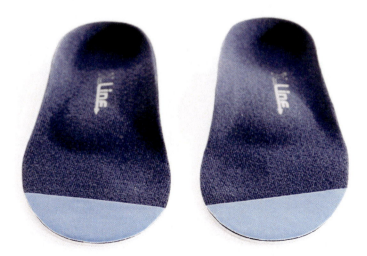

Figure 51: Rectangle ENGO patch (with excess trimmed off) providing a low-friction surface for the tips of clawed or hammer toes.

5 Silicone gel toe caps

Silicone gel toe caps are closed in at the end and work by cushioning and absorbing shear at the tip of the toes. Consider these once you have dealt with your nails appropriately and if you have adequate room in your shoe. Without these prerequisites in place you'll probably still get blisters. Also be wary of skin maceration as the silicone gel material prevents sweat from evaporating. The extent to which this is a problem depends on the individual, so experiment with them.

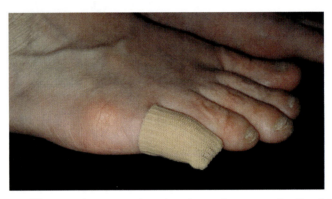

Figure 52: Silicone gel toe cap, closed at the end to cover the tip of the toe.

6 Alter your biomechanics

Some people have a hyperextended interphalangeal joint of the big toe (pictured below). This "cocked-up" big toe results in the end of the toe (and therefore the nail) pointing upwards rather than being parallel with the floor. If the shoe is not deep enough in the toe box the toenail gets pressure from the top of the shoe and is pushed back into the toe with each step – ouch!

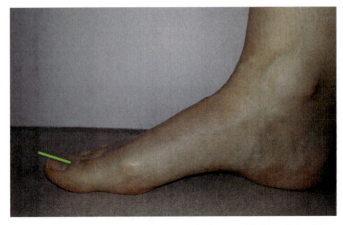

Figure 53: A mildmoderate hyperextended interphalangeal joint of the big toe caused the nail to be angled upwards.

This cocked-up position is a common consequence of the big toe knuckle being stiff - which is often caused by an inefficient windlass mechanism.

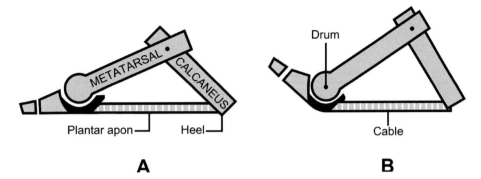

Figure 54: The Windlass Mechanism. If the big toe is unable to roll up on the knuckle (drum), the joint in the middle of the big toe can become hyperextended, making the end of the toe angle upwards.

Fixing this depends on whether the stiffness is a functional or a structural stiffness.

- A functional stiffness can be helped by a podiatrist. Depending on your mechanics, this may involve orthotics (with specific additions for the functional hallux limitus issue), heel lifts, calf stretches or a few other modalities, all aimed at improving windlass mechanism function. Have a look at the image below. To start with, the toe is cocked-up at the end making the toenail angle upwards. But a piece of material under the first bone of the toe makes it sit more parallel with the floor. This is just one example of what a podiatrist can do to change your foot mechanics to help you prevent toenail blisters of the big toe.

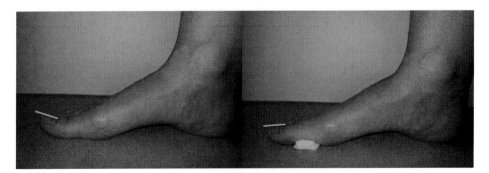

Figure 55: Big toe cocked-up. Note the angle of the toenail. A podiatrist can use one of many treatments to encourage the toe to sit straighter.

- A structural (bony) stiffness is not so easy to resolve. Talk to your podiatrist about the options such as different types of orthotics, footwear modifications, and surgery if it's a big enough problem for you. Or do what you can to get shoes that are really deep in the toe box to accommodate it. This can be easier said than done. Ladies, consider buying men's runners - they are a bit deeper for the length.

7 Change the terrain or your technique

Running or walking downhill causes your foot to move forward in the shoe with more force. That means you're more likely to get toenail blisters going downhill than if you were on the flat or going uphill.

Assuming you can't change the terrain you're on, changing your technique in one of the following ways could help.

- A shorter stride length;
- More knee and hip flexion; or
- If your initial ground contact when running is a forefoot strike, try and get a bit of heel strike or at least midfoot strike.

Remember, making sudden changes to your gait can cause injury. Introduce changes in speed, duration and technique gradually.

Summary

If you're blister prone …
If you're very active and struggling with foot blisters …
If you've tried a number of things and they don't work …
It's time to take a different approach.

Preventing blisters can be easy.
But you need to consider each anatomical location on its own merits.
This is what it takes to get on top of blisters when basic blister prevention techniques fail.

This book lays the foundations.
Consider how these strategies could work for your feet and for your blisters.
Get help where you need it. And enjoy a new sensation, your new reality …

Being blister-free!

Glossary

Biomechanics: The study of the mechanical laws relating to the movement and structure of living organisms, particularly of the forces exerted by muscles and gravity on the skeleton.

Gait: Walking or running technique

Shear: The stretching and distortion of skin and soft tissue between skin and bone. The cause of blisters.

Windlass mechanism: The functional shortening of the plantarfascia between the calcaneus and metatarsals as the big toe rolls up on the metatarsal head. This winding of the plantarfascia shortens the distance between the calcaneus and metatarsals to elevate the medial longitudinal arch, preparing the foot for effective propulsion.

About the author

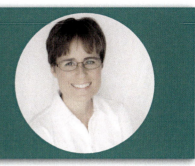

Rebecca Rushton BSc(Pod) graduated from Curtin University, Perth, Western Australia in 1993. She works in private practice at Esperance Podiatry and enjoys living in one of the most beautiful and pristine parts of the world. Every now and then, Rebecca ventures out of Esperance to help athletes manage their blisters, providing specialist foot care at multiday ultramarathons.

Rebecca has a personal and professional special interest in foot blisters. In 2012, she founded *Blister Prevention*, an online resource for athletes and sports medicine professionals requiring information about foot blister management. And she is the Australian distributor for ENGO Blister Patches. Her work at Blister Prevention has seen Rebecca become an authority on the subject. She wrote *The Advanced Guide to Blister Prevention*, which has been described as "an incredible resource on this often trivialised foot injury" by Simon Bartold of Bartold Biomechanics.

Questions? Comments?

Help make the next edition of this book even better. Email suggestions to support@blisterprevention.com.au

Need help?

I help health professionals, athletes and everyday people all around the world with blisters. From free resources to online consulting and providing foot care at races. For more information, visit my website at www.blisterprevention.com.au.

Rebecca Rushton

Made in the USA
Las Vegas, NV
05 February 2025

17609625R00036